# Stretching for Seniors

Exercises and Stretches for Improving Strength, Flexibility and Balance to Remain Stable and Free of Pain in the Golden Years

By Milton Davy

*Self Puplished ?*

© Copyright 2020 - All rights reserved.

The content contained within this book may not be reproduced, duplicated or transmitted without direct written permission from the author or the publisher.

Under no circumstances will any blame or legal responsibility be held against the publisher or author for any damages, reparation, or monetary loss due to the information contained within this book. Either directly or indirectly.

Legal Notice:

This book is copyright protected. This book is only for personal use. You cannot amend, distribute, sell, use, quote or paraphrase any part, or the content within this book, without the consent of the author or publisher.

Disclaimer Notice:

Please note the information contained within this document is for educational and entertainment purposes only. All effort has been executed to present accurate, up to date and reliable, complete information. No warranties of any kind are declared or implied. Readers acknowledge that the author is not engaging in the rendering of legal, financial, medical or professional advice. The content within this book has been derived from various sources. Please consult a licensed professional before attempting any techniques outlined in this book.

By reading this document, the reader agrees that under no circumstances is the author responsible for any losses, direct or indirect, which are incurred as a result of the use of information contained within this document, including, but not limited to, —errors, omissions, or inaccuracies.

# Contents

Introduction ..................................................................................... 1
   Muscle and Bone Issues in the Aging Body ........................... 2
   Changes in the Muscles ......................................................... 2
   Changes in the Bones ............................................................ 3
   Changes in the Joints ............................................................ 3
   How This Book Can Assist You ............................................... 4

Chapter 1: Fundamental Anatomy ................................................. 5
   Primary Muscle Groups ......................................................... 5
   Primary Joints ....................................................................... 8

Chapter 2-- Why is Stretching Good ............................................. 10
   Muscles and Stretching ....................................................... 10
   Bones and Stretching .......................................................... 11
   Joints and Stretching .......................................................... 12
   Other Health Advantages ................................................... 13

Chapter 3-- Things to Think About Beforehand ........................... 14
   Speak to Your Physician ...................................................... 14
   Locate a Trainer .................................................................. 15
   Find a Location ................................................................... 15
   Have Correct Clothes .......................................................... 16
   Get Some Stretching Tools ................................................. 16

Chapter 4-- Kinds Of Stretches ..................................................... 18
   Ballistic Stretching .............................................................. 18
   Active Stretching ................................................................ 19
   Passive Stretching .............................................................. 19

- Isometric Stretching.................................................................19
- Dynamic Stretching..................................................................20
- PNF Stretching........................................................................20
- Timing of Stretches.................................................................21

## Chapter 5 - Stretch Training Programs ...............................22
- Yoga ........................................................................................22
- Benefits of Yoga .....................................................................22
- Disadvantages of Yoga ..........................................................23
- Pilates .....................................................................................24
- Benefits of Pilates ..................................................................24
- Disadvantages of Pilates ......................................................24

## Chapter 6 -- Typical Stumbling Blocks to Stretch Training & Dangers .....26
- No Time ..................................................................................26
- Movement Hurts ...................................................................27
- No Energy ...............................................................................27
- Not Warming Up....................................................................28
- Inappropriate Stretches........................................................28
- Falling......................................................................................29

## Chapter 7 -- Stretch Workouts for Novices ........................30
- Warmup..................................................................................30
- Stretch Workout ....................................................................31
- When to Cool off ...................................................................32

## Chapter 8 -- Sample Stretch Workouts................................34
- Targeting Muscle Groups......................................................36
- Targeting Joints.....................................................................37

## Chapter 9 - Tools/Apps/Resources .......................................38

- Foam Roller ........................................................................... 38
- Lacrosse Ball ........................................................................ 39
- Rope ...................................................................................... 39
- Classes ................................................................................. 39
- Personal Trainer/Physical Therapist .................................. 40
- Apps ..................................................................................... 40

## Conclusion-- Tips to Include Stretching into Your Life ........... 42
- Have a Schedule ................................................................. 43
- Utilize Friends and Family ................................................. 43
- Sign Up With an Online Community ................................. 44
- Have a Calendar ................................................................. 45
- Give Yourself a Reward ..................................................... 45

## Bonus Chapter-- Advanced Stretch Workouts ......................... 47
- Yoga Positions .................................................................... 47
- Pilates .................................................................................. 48
- Active Stretching ................................................................ 48
- Dynamic Stretching ........................................................... 49
- Utilizing Tools .................................................................... 49

Thank you for buying this book and I hope that you will find it useful. If you will want to share your thoughts on this book, you can do so by leaving a review on the Amazon page, it helps me out a lot.

# Introduction

Hey there, and welcome to this book on stretching methods to keep steady & loose for seniors.

As you grow older, your body is going to undergo a great deal of alterations. Your hair is going to turn white or grey, your skin is going to end up being wrinkly and old, and your body is going to end up being stiff as you experience muscle, joint and bone issues. For several years, we have actually accepted that tensing of the joints and tightening up of the muscles are normal parts of aging. However, brand-new research proposes otherwise.

Research has actually now discovered that at least half of the alterations aging individuals experience in regards to their muscles, joints and bones are due to an absence of activity.

Nevertheless, when less than 10 percent of individuals over the age of 50 aren't getting ample physical exercise to preserve their health at the very least, it's not surprising that a lot of individuals have actually accepted their fates.

## Muscle and Bone Issues in the Aging Body

The most typical muscle and bone issues the aging body might experience consist of osteoarthritis when the cartilage in your joints starts to deteriorate, osteomalacia which is a softening of the bones, osteoporosis that causes fragile bones when bones lose their mass, rheumatoid arthritis that is a swelling in the joints, and overall muscle discomfort and weakness.

## Changes in the Muscles

As we grow older, there are a couple of alterations that our muscles undergo that result in the above issues. Our muscle fibers become tinier and we have less of them, and nerve system alterations result in less muscle tone and a reduced capability to contract muscles. Lost muscle tissue is restored more gradually than previously, and the tissue that substitutes it is typically hard and fibrous.

## Changes in the Bones

We do not typically consider bones as living tissue, however, they definitely are, and additionally undergo alterations as we age. Our bones start to lose more calcium and other crucial minerals due to the hormonal alterations that take place as we age. Ladies are particularly susceptible after they have actually undergone menopause, however, males are additionally impacted by bone loss that accompanies age.

## Changes in the Joints

The motion in our joints is an outcome of the motion of ligaments, the streaming of synovial fluid that encompasses your joints, and layers of cartilage that prevents bones from coming into straight contact with one another. Nevertheless, in the aging body, ligaments can end up being much shorter and less pliable since there is less synovial fluid to grease the joints and cartilage thins. All of this causes tensing in the joints.

## How This Book Can Assist You

A surprising amount of these age-related conditions could be reversed or avoided via routine exercise and stretching. This book particularly concentrates on how to utilize stretching as a method to keep flexibility and limberness regardless of how old you are. The reality is, it's never ever too late to begin doing something for your body.

By the conclusion of this book, you are going to have all the tools you require to maintain your body in the best attainable shape so that you can delight in your golden years.

## Chapter 1: Fundamental Anatomy

The main objective of stretching the aging body is to stop muscles and joints from ending up being stiff from disuse. By routinely stretching your muscles and flexing your joints, you can assist in protecting against much of the age-related ailments that impact the muscles, joints and bones of an aging body. In this part of the book, we will look at the primary muscle groups and joints that need to be kept limber.

**Primary Muscle Groups**

There are 11 primary muscle groups that you wish to make certain you're utilizing routinely. If you are additionally performing strength training exercises, these are the identical muscle groups that you are going to be exercising with that.

Forearms-- Your lower arm has a number of muscles that are especially crucial for raising and holding things.

Biceps-- A big muscle located on each of your upper arms, your biceps assist your forearms with raising objects.

Triceps-- These are the other 2 muscles that are located on your upper arms. They assist your body to bend and extend your elbows.

Shoulders-- There are a variety of muscles on your back, front and the side that comprise the shoulders which are in charge of arm motion.

Trapezius-- Typically referred to as traps. These are the muscles in your upper back that assist with moving your head, neck and shoulder blade.

Chest-- This group of muscles that encompasses your ribcage is in charge of assisting with breathing and arm motion.

Abdominals-- This crucial group of muscles found in your abdominal area aids with breathing and supports your spinal column. They are frequently referred to as your core muscles or abs.

Back-- Among the largest muscle groups, your back muscles assist in supporting your spinal column and your hip motion.

Quadriceps-- These are the 4 muscles that are located at the front of your thigh and are an important part of leg motion as they assist in managing the knee and hip motions.

Hamstrings-- The group of muscles that comprises the back of your thigh and aids with the motion of the knee and the hips too.

Calves-- The muscles located in your lower leg are what assist you with moving your knee and flexing your ankle.

## Primary Joints

Even though you have a variety of tinier joints in your toes and fingers, there are 7 primary joints in the remainder of your body that we're going to go over. Every joint is comprised of a mix of muscles that enable the motion, tendons and ligaments that link bones, along with bones and muscles.

**Spinal column**-- Your spinal column assists with supporting your upper body and houses the nerves that go to every system in the body. It's comprised of a variety of vertebrae.

**Shoulder**-- Mostly in charge of arm motions.

**Elbow**-- At the center of your arm, it aids with lifting.

**Wrist**-- Comprised of a variety of parts, your wrist is a vital part of hand motion.

Hip-- Another ball-and-socket joint, this one is in charge of entire leg motions.

Knee-- This leg joint assists you with walking.

Ankle-- Another joint that has numerous parts, your ankle supports your legs and aids with walking.

In the following part, we'll be diving more into the science of why stretching these muscle groups can aid with the aging body.

## Chapter 2-- Why is Stretching Good

As we went over previously, there are a variety of issues with our muscles, joints, and bones that we deal with as our body ages. Luckily, there is something that we may do about it, which is stretching. Stretching in addition to other exercises can assist in preventing and even reversing a number of the issues we talked about previously.

### Muscles and Stretching

When you're not utilizing your muscles enough, they can end up being stiff, which causes unpleasant motions. By frequently stretching, you can prevent your muscles from getting stiff and you can enhance their flexibility. The more flexible your muscles are, the less discomfort you are going to experience when you set about your day, and the more you are going to have the ability to do.

Another advantage of routinely stretching your aging muscles is that it is going to enhance your balance. This is due to the fact that when your muscles are frequently stretched, they can respond much better to movements, which assists you with remaining well balanced. This is going to enable you to be more self-assured when carrying out other exercises along with protecting against falls, which are specifically unsafe for the aging body.

**Bones and Stretching**

While stretching itself does not bolster your bones, a variety of exercises do, featuring walking, which you have to do prior to each stretching session to warm your muscles up. In case you have particular worries about bone loss, you are going to wish to make certain you are doing some easy exercises that can develop bone mass along with stretching exercises.

Furthermore, by stretching routinely, you are going to develop the range of movement in your joints and much better muscle flexibility, which is going to assist you in doing the exercises that you have to do to enhance your bone health. As your muscles move and get sturdier throughout the exercise, your bones are going to gain back the bone density that was lost as you grew older.

## Joints and Stretching

Stretching can assist in making your joints more flexible, which is essential for aging bodies, given that joints have a tendency to get stiffer with age. With higher flexibility, you have a much better range of movement. This can assist in getting rid of motions that were formerly unpleasant, consisting of numerous kinds of exercise and day-to-day activities.

Another advantage of stretching is the stretching of tendons. Tendons link your muscles to your bones and can get stiff and shorten when they are not utilized. The very best method to extend and loosen up your tendons to get your joints moving well once again is by frequently stretching.

The other part of the joints are the ligaments that hold bones together. These are meant to be hard and not really versatile due to the fact that they offer stability in the joint. Nevertheless, with age, they can end up being too rigid, so stretching is going to assist in getting them back to where they're meant to be. So, instead of limiting your motions, they support your joints and enable you to move easily.

**Other Health Advantages**

There are numerous other health advantages to stretching, like assisting you to unwind, enhancing your posture, boosting energy levels, promoting blood flow, and decreasing cholesterol. Keep going through this book to discover more about how to stretch your aging body to enhance your wellbeing.

## Chapter 3-- Things to Think About Beforehand

Prior to beginning with a stretching program, it is essential that you do these things initially. Despite the fact that it might appear easy to start stretching frequently, if you are not effectively prepared, you have a much greater threat of injury. Preparation is going to additionally assist you with understanding precisely what you are getting involved in so you can adhere to the program you choose.

### Speak to Your Physician

Speaking to your physician about your present health is the most vital thing that you may do prior to beginning a stretching program. They are going to have the ability to tell you what areas you have to concentrate on and how frequently you ought to stretch to enhance your health. In case you have issues with your heart or bones, they might additionally put you on supplements or medications.

## Locate a Trainer

If you are brand-new to stretching or your physician advises that you collaborate with someone to concentrate on particular issues, then you are going to have to locate a trainer. For assistance with stretching, you might participate in classes or locate somebody through a neighborhood gym. Nevertheless, if you have physical constraints, you might want to locate a physiotherapist to assist you.

## Find a Location

It's advised to locate a location where you may do your stretching workouts most conveniently and successfully. You might select to do this at home, a gym, or your neighborhood community center. Considering that some stretches need some extra tools, you'll want to ensure you have access to these anywhere you are. Lots of community centers are going to have little workout centers that are ideal for carrying out workouts, and they are typically far more budget-friendly than gyms.

## Have Correct Clothes

Donning the appropriate clothes can assist you to stretch far more easily, however, it does not need to be anything lavish or too costly, so do not worry. You should wear clothes that will not limit your motions by any means. This could be tight-fitting clothes like yoga pants or spandex.

## Get Some Stretching Tools

You may do numerous stretches without tools, however, having some standard tools is going to make some stretches safer and easier for your aging body. Resistance bands or stretch bands are excellent for making numerous stretches simpler and more powerful. An incline board offers you with an angled surface area for numerous leg stretches, and a yoga mat is ideal for cushioning your body when performing any stretches from the floor.

There are additionally a variety of devices created particularly for stretching. These are an excellent way to get going since they push you to do the stretch appropriately, which assists with avoiding injury while enhancing the effectiveness of the stretch. Sadly, these are usually relatively pricey, so if you can discover a gym that has them, that is usually a much better alternative.

When you have all the things prepared, the only thing left to do is to keep reading to find out more about stretching to get going with stretching daily.

## Chapter 4-- Kinds Of Stretches

In this part of the book, we're going to look at the various kinds of stretches that are performed and which kind of stretching is going to be ideal for you and your aging body. We'll additionally speak about why timing stretches is essential, and we will go over just how much time you need for each stretch.

### Ballistic Stretching

If you have actually ever seen anybody bouncing while stretching, this is ballistic stretching. The concept is that it utilizes the momentum of your motion to press a joint beyond its regular range of motion.

This is one kind that you ought to stay clear of at all costs as it can typically induce your muscles to get tighter, and it can even induce injury.

### Active Stretching

Typically utilized in yoga, this entails bringing your limb into position with no assistance from props or other limbs and letting just the muscles in that limb to hold the stretch. This could be exceptionally challenging, which is why it's hardly ever held for more than 10 seconds at once. However, it's terrific for building muscle.

### Passive Stretching

Like active stretching, passive stretching has you presuming and keeping a position. Nevertheless, these stretches are held for a lot longer time period (1 minute or more) due to the fact that they utilize props that enable you to keep the stretch. These are excellent for injuries as they do not work the muscles too much.

### Isometric Stretching

This kind of stretching entails utilizing your own strength to press past the passive stretch. You presume a position, and after that, press versus the prop (or your trainer sometimes) to produce a much deeper stretch on those muscles, which is a terrific method to involve more of your muscle fibers than passive stretching alone.

**Dynamic Stretching.**

This is another kind of stretching that entails motion, and it is secure and helpful. With dynamic stretching, you carry out sets of particular leg and arm motions that enable your joints to carefully and naturally extend beyond their previous limitations, exercising them and bending the muscles simultaneously.

**PNF Stretching.**

PNF means proprioceptive neuromuscular facilitation, and it basically utilizes a mix of isometric and passive stretches to supply even better outcomes. Due to the mix of stretches, this is the fastest method to enhance versatility via stretching.

## Timing of Stretches.

As we pointed out, various stretches are held for various quantities of time. This is, in some cases, related to the challenge of the stretch as with dynamic and active stretches, however, the usefulness of the stretch is additionally a variable. Although an active stretch might just need 10 seconds to be useful, doing a passive stretch for identical quantity of time would not produce any outcomes.

Given that many isometric and passive stretches need at least one minute for every one of the primary muscles, you'll want to make certain that you provide yourself with a lot of time for every stretching session. Enabling your muscles to stretch for a minimum of a minute each provides an opportunity to slowly stretch out and keep that position for enough time to affect that muscle for more than a handful of minutes after your session.

## Chapter 5 - Stretch Training Programs

When it pertains to stretch training, there are 2 kinds of programs that are most prominent: Pilates and yoga. However, prior to registering for the next class being offered in your location, we will discuss just what these stretch training programs are and assist you in identifying how helpful they are for you and your aging body.

### Yoga

Yoga emerged as a spiritual discipline established by Hindus to integrate meditation, breathing control, and various body postures to make spiritual connections. Now, you can discover lots of people who focus just on the health advantages of yoga, which utilizes both passive and active stretches.

### Benefits of Yoga

A few of the benefits of doing yoga routinely consist of boosted strength and flexibility, enhanced blood circulation, and stress relief. Even though there are definitely some challenging postures, a seasoned trainer can assist you in carrying out customized variations of these or assist you in discovering postures that you may do that provide you with the identical stretch.

Disadvantages of Yoga

Bikram or Hot Yoga is something you ought to stay clear of since there is proof that this could be unsafe for your health. However, beyond that, the greatest downside to yoga is getting an instructor that presses you too hard, which can induce you to hurt yourself while attempting something you should not have actually been carrying out in the first place.

Bottom line: Yoga is a terrific method to enhance flexibility and strength, however, you want to ensure you have a great trainer who is going to assist you in achieving your objectives and will not place your aging body at risk of injury.

## Pilates

Pilates is a kind of exercise that integrates a mix of floor exercises and specialized devices to enhance flexibility and strength. It particularly concentrates on reinforcing your core muscles and mostly utilizes isotonic and dynamic stretches in addition to different exercises.

### Benefits of Pilates

Pilates benefits the aging body due to the fact that it enhances the muscles, specifically the core, which results in much better posture and balance, and it increases versatility and variety of movement. It can additionally be simpler for novices and could be quickly personalized to assist with rehabilitating particular injuries.

### Disadvantages of Pilates

A few of the downsides of Pilates are that it will not assist with weight reduction, the motions need a good deal of concentration to carry out properly, progress is tough to track which makes it difficult to understand how far you have actually come, and if you do have a particular concern, it could be difficult to get the personal attention you require in a class setting.

Bottom line: Pilates could be a terrific method to be being more versatile and to boost your physical strength, but for individuals with physical restrictions, it might be difficult to discover a perfect setting in which their issues could be appropriately dealt with.

Final word: Both Pilates and yoga could be helpful for the aging body, however, not everyone can walk into any Pilates or yoga class, so take your time and discover the best one.

# Chapter 6-- Typical Stumbling Blocks to Stretch Training & Dangers

There are a variety of stumbling blocks that can keep individuals from stretch training along with a couple of risks that you want to be knowledgeable about prior to starting. Initially, we're going to take a look at a few of the important things that might be keeping you from doing stretch training and show you some easy methods to conquer them.

## No Time

Many individuals feel that they just do not have time to do stretch exercises since it does take a while to make certain all of your muscles have actually been correctly stretched. Nevertheless, if you take a closer look at your schedule, you might discover some big chunks of time while watching television. Combine this time with your stretch training, and you will not get bored throughout the stretching.

## Movement Hurts

It could be difficult to wish to stretch your muscles and move your joints when they hurt, so bear in mind that what you're doing is going to assist with removing this discomfort with time. You can additionally customize the majority of stretches to ensure that they're not unpleasant while they are still helpful. When you're beginning, make certain not to overdo it. Take things slowly and progress at your own speed.

## No Energy

I absolutely understand that your aging body does not have as much energy as it once did, however, do not allow that to stop you from doing what's ideal for your body. Stretch training is easy on your body and can, in fact, make you feel more invigorated as it enhances blood flow that can assist you to feel more awake and alert.

Now, let's take a look at a few of the risks of stretch training that you want to be knowledgeable about.

## Not Warming Up

Picture your muscles like an elastic band. If you attempt to stretch them when they're cold, they're likely to tear and even snap in half. However, if you warm them up initially, then they will have the ability to stretch further and will not break. Similarly, if you leap right into isotonic or passive stretches without warming your muscles up, you might quickly harm your muscles.

## Inappropriate Stretches

In case you move your limb the wrong way throughout stretch training, you can place excessive pressure on the muscle or the joint, which can result in an injury. This is why it's ideal for somebody who has actually never ever frequently done stretch training to locate a trainer that can assist them in discovering the proper method to stretch to avoid this danger.

# Falling

This is a typical worry about the aging body as falls are riskier and more likely as your balance can end up being impaired with age. Even though this is a genuine threat throughout stretch training as some stretches do need balance, there are a lot of things that you may do to decrease this danger, like utilizing a wall or chair for assistance or cooperating with a strong partner who can assist you.

# Chapter 7-- Stretch Workouts for Novices

In this part of the book, I will provide you with an overview of a stretch workout, that has 2 standard parts: the stretching and the warmup. Although many workouts need a cooldown stage after the main part of your workout, you can skip that with stretch training since it does not work your muscles hard enough.

**Warmup**

As discussed in the last part, stretching your muscles without warming up can cause injuries and muscle tears, which is why it's so essential to take a minimum of 10 minutes to get your body prepared to stretch. Thankfully, warming up is extremely simple to do, and the physical activity is additionally terrific for enhancing muscle strength and blood flow.

The simplest warmup for a stretch regimen is walking for 10 minutes. If you are performing your stretch training in your house, you can walk up and down the corridor, and you can even walk in place.

Since you are going to additionally be stretching your arm muscles, it is essential to move your arms more than you usually would during walking, as if you were running in slow motion.

Stretch Workout

Throughout your stretch workout, you are going to have to work through all the primary muscle groups to make certain you cover all of them. Once again, the 11 primary muscle groups are: biceps, forearms, triceps, trapezius, shoulders, abdominals, chest, back, hamstrings, quadriceps, and calves. Whether you utilize the stretch regimen from the next part or develop your own, make sure to cover all of the primary muscle groups.

It's additionally essential to utilize different kinds of stretches. Active and dynamic stretches are excellent for enhancing muscle strength which is additionally great for enhancing bone mass, so you might wish to attempt these if you worry about bone loss. Isotonic and passive stretches are a lot easier to perform and are much better for individuals who are concerned about having the ability to balance.

Make certain to perform each stretch for the length of time that is suggested for that stretch. There is a reason why you ought to perform that stretch for that long, and even though it most likely will not hurt to perform it for longer, if you perform it for a shorter quantity of time, it will not be nearly as helpful because you will not get the outcomes you're after.

Another thing to bear in mind throughout a stretch workout is that stretching must not hurt. You ought to feel the muscle stretching, and you might experience some moderate discomfort, however, in case you experience pain in your muscles, this is an indication that you are either performing the stretch incorrectly or are pressing yourself too far, too quick, and have to work your way up to stretching that far.

When to Cool off

If you do decide to perform dynamic stretching, you might benefit from a light cooldown. This can include merely walking for 10 minutes and/or performing a couple of isotonic or passive stretches to assist your muscles to totally unwind after your stretch regimen.

## Chapter 8-- Sample Stretch Workouts

In this part, I will offer you a list of the very best stretches for each of the 11 groups of muscles. You can utilize these for your stretch workout, or discover ones that are simpler for you to perform for every muscle group. Prior to starting, warm up for a minimum of 10 minutes, so your muscles are prepared to be stretched. You additionally wish to ensure that you hold every stretch for 30 seconds to 1 minute.

Forearm-- The most effective stretches for the forearm are the standing wrist flexor stretch, standing extensor stretch, wrist rotations, and assisted forearm stretch.

Biceps-- For your biceps, you are going to wish to attempt the biceps wall stretch, standing biceps stretch, doorway biceps stretch, wrist-rotation biceps stretch, and seated bent-knee biceps stretch.

Triceps-- To stretch out your triceps, utilize the crossbody triceps stretch and the overhead triceps stretch.

Shoulder-- To enhance versatility in your shoulders, you'll wish to perform neck rolls, chin retractions, shoulder rotation, shoulder rolls, and the standing wall stretch.

Trapezius-- The most effective stretches to relax your trapezius muscles are the side trapezius stretch, forward trapezius stretch, and diagonal trapezius stretch.

Chest-- To stretch your chest, you'll want to perform the elbow wrap stretch, wall stretch, lying chest stretch, back bend stretch, and the standing chest expansion.

Abdominals-- For your abdominal muscles, you'll wish to perform the standing abdominal stretch, lying abdominal stretch, and abdominal rotations.

**Back**-- To stretch your back muscles, you'll wish to attempt the lying knee twist, knee to chest stretch, piriformis seated stretch, and yoga positions like the restful post, cobra, and the cat/cow positions.

**Quadriceps**-- There are 3 stretches that are fantastic for the quadriceps: standing quadriceps stretch, the kneeling quadriceps stretch, and ground quadriceps stretch.

**Hamstrings**-- A few of the most effective stretches for the hamstrings are the hamstring twist, hamstring slider, butterfly, modified hamstring twist, single-leg circle, and open-air stretch.

**Calves**-- The most effective muscles for your calves are wall calf stretch, the standing calf stretch, and the downward dog yoga pose.

### Targeting Muscle Groups

To target particular muscle groups that are especially aching or stiff, then you might have to perform a number of sets of stretches for those muscles. You might additionally think about holding every stretch for as much as 3 minutes each to enable more of your muscle fibers inside that muscle to have time to be stretched out. You can additionally perform these stretching exercises more than once daily to assist with enhancing flexibility quicker.

**Targeting Joints**

If you have a specific joint that you wish to boost your range of motion in, then you are going to want to concentrate on the muscle groups that manage that joint. Consider what muscles are on either side of that joint and perform more stretches in those muscles. For instance, if your knees are an issue, then you are going to wish to stretch your hamstrings, quadriceps, and calves more than other muscles.

## Chapter 9 - Tools/Apps/Resources

If you believe that remaining loose into older age is going to be challenging, then make sure to use these tools, apps, and resources that are going to assist you in reaching your flexibility objectives. Make sure to utilize the tools that are going to be most helpful for you personally when it concerns stretch training, considering that not every one of the resources is going to be best for each individual.

### Foam Roller

Among the very best tools you can purchase that are going to assist you with your stretch training is a foam roller. Since it's so helpful, it can additionally hurt, specifically when you're initially utilizing it. Nevertheless, if you desire excellent outcomes, especially in your calves and back, this is an excellent tool to have. To effectively discover how to utilize one and which type is ideal for you, you might want to work with a trainer or participate in a foam roller class.

### Lacrosse Ball

Another practical tool you might think about purchasing is a lacrosse ball. These enable you to carry out self-massage in the spots that require some additional assistance, such as the back or neck. A lacrosse ball allows you to put pressure in a specific area where you might have connective tissues bunched up in knots. Working on these knotted fibers is going to assist you to feel much better while being more mobile.

### Rope

You can additionally utilize a piece of rope or perhaps a towel to assist with offering resistance for isotonic stretches. Having a number of towels or ropes of various lengths is going to assist you to enhance the effectiveness of your stretches.

### Classes

There are various classes that you can take that can assist by means of neighborhood community of like-minded individuals that supply you with a certified trainer that can instruct you on how to appropriately stretch without hurting yourself. Take some time to discover a class that is best for you, and do not hesitate to ask if you can take one class to give it a try

Personal Trainer/Physical Therapist

If you have a particular health issue that requires attention, you might have to work individually with a personal trainer or a physiotherapist that can ensure the stretches you're doing are going to, in fact, assist you instead of making things worse. Your physician can typically advise a great physiotherapist, and numerous fitness centers have personal trainers that can assist.

Apps

Phone apps are another excellent method to assist you to adhere to your stretching regimen. Some exercise apps are going to even allow you to come up with your own exercise program where you can include stretches and set the length of time you wish to do every one. Then, when you're prepared to stretch, all you need to do is begin the workout while following the instructions.

By utilizing a mix of these resources, you can keep yourself on course with your stretch training system and achieve success. In the next part, I'll offer you additional ideas that you can utilize to make stretching part of your day-to-day regimen.

## Conclusion-- Tips to Include Stretching into Your Life

Congratulations on making it to the conclusion of this guide, which is about showing you how you can remain loose and steady as a senior. You might be amazed to know that most of the individuals who start something never ever finish it.

Take your time and progress at your own pace. This is not a race. The more you comprehend and understand what is occurring when you carry out a stretching & stability course, the better.

If you truly wish to prosper, then everything you do for your body needs to be with long-term organization in mind. These modifications you're making and the diet plan you're following are not implied to be short-term solutions. They're meant to be part of a brand-new way of life that you stick to in order to keep off the weight that you lost while maintaining your health.

Equally as crucial as performing the stretches correctly is doing them daily, which is why in this part, I will provide you with some pointers that you can utilize to include stretching into your everyday life so you can stay with it and continue reaping the benefits of a stretch system.

## Have a Schedule

Prior to beginning with your stretch training regimen, you wish to identify precisely when you will do it. If you're stressed, you'll get too occupied throughout the day and forget about stretching. You might wish to do your stretching first thing in the early morning. If you understand that you'll have much better luck after lunch or right prior to bed, then set aside that time for stretch training and do not allow anything else to hamper it.

## Utilize Friends and Family

Among the very best methods to assist with keeping you on course with your stretch training is utilizing individuals around you. If you can discover a stretching partner, it could be an enjoyable method to hang out together and to keep one another accountable to ensure you're stretching as frequently as you need to. It can additionally be a good idea to carry out these stretches with somebody else to assist you.

Doing things such as posting about your workout on Facebook is another method to get excellent support from your friends and family. In case you make a dedication to publish about your workout daily or to let someone know when you finish your stretch workout, then you can remain accountable, and you are going to get lots of support.

**Sign Up With an Online Community**

There are lots of online communities that you can sign up with that are going to assist you to remain on course with your stretch training. These are additionally fantastic places to ask questions about what you're doing so that you can get pointers on how to get the most out of your stretch training. When searching for an excellent online community to sign up with, make certain to take a look at how active and reliable the members are.

## Have a Calendar

Having a calendar where you note the days on which you performed your stretch training is an excellent way to remind yourself that you have to do it daily and an excellent way to keep yourself accountable. You can mark days merely by placing a large happy face on the calendar when you're finished for the day.

## Give Yourself a Reward

Rewarding yourself is an excellent method to utilize positive reinforcement to keep yourself on course. It might be that you offer yourself a little healthy reward at the conclusion of each training session, or that you enable yourself to purchase something particular at the conclusion of a week if you trained every day. Make certain that whatever you pick as your reward, it is a thing that won't harm your health.

By making stretch training a priority, you are going to see the favorable outcomes from it that you're after!

## Bonus Chapter-- Advanced Stretch Workouts

When you have actually mastered the fundamentals of the passive stretches noted previously, you'll wish to start with more advanced stretch workouts. Advanced stretch workouts are going to enable you to transcend where you are now and assist you in pressing yourself to be a lot more versatile. Make certain to include advanced stretches to your regimen gradually, so you do not hurt yourself.

### Yoga Positions

There are a variety of yoga positions that ought to just be done by somebody who has actually totally mastered the fundamentals of stretching. In case you are taking yoga classes as your primary kind of stretch training, you ought to constantly begin with a novice class or one developed particularly for the aging body. Your instructor can inform you when you are prepared to attempt a more advanced class.

Pilates

Due to the fact that Pilates entails a variety of motions along with stretches, it's not for everybody, however it is terrific for developing strength in muscles together with versatility. Lots of Pilates moves could be performed at home with nothing but a yoga mat, however there are lots of others that need customized tools. Luckily, you can discover Pilates classes that have what you require: qualified instructors and special equipment.

Active Stretching

Instead of doing just passive stretching, you'll wish to include active stretching to your arsenal. These stretches are far tougher due to the fact that you need to utilize the muscle to hold your limb in place. This is what makes them perfect for developing strength, together with versatility. Due to the fact that active stretching utilizes the muscles, you are going to most likely have to cool off after a stretching session with some light walking.

Dynamic Stretching

In case you have issues with balance, be extremely careful when doing dynamic stretching as it entails a great deal of motion, typically one leg at once. Although you ought to be utilizing a wall or sturdy chair for assistance, this might be challenging for individuals with balance issues. Nevertheless, if you can include these to your regimen, dynamic stretches are terrific for enhancing versatility and muscle strength simultaneously.

Utilizing Tools

I have actually pointed out a couple of tools throughout the book that you can utilize to enhance your stretch training. We have actually talked about resistance or stretch bands, lacrosse balls, yoga mats, incline boards, foam rollers, stretch machines, and a rope or towel. All of these things are made to assist you to stretch much better

You are going to likely wish to just include a couple of these things at once, so check out each stretch training tool to see what would work ideally for you as far as targeting particular issues or muscle groups. Then, when you have actually mastered using one tool, you can include another one up until you have everything you feel you require for your stretch training requirements.

Thank you for putting in the time to go through this book on stretching for the aging body. I hope that you have all the information you require to be able to remain loose even as time appears to be working against you. By being consistent and utilizing all of your resources intelligently, you can keep your joints and muscles loose regardless of how old you are.

I hope that you enjoyed reading through this book and that you have found it useful. If you want to share your thoughts on this book, you can do so by leaving a review on the Amazon page. Have a great rest of the day.

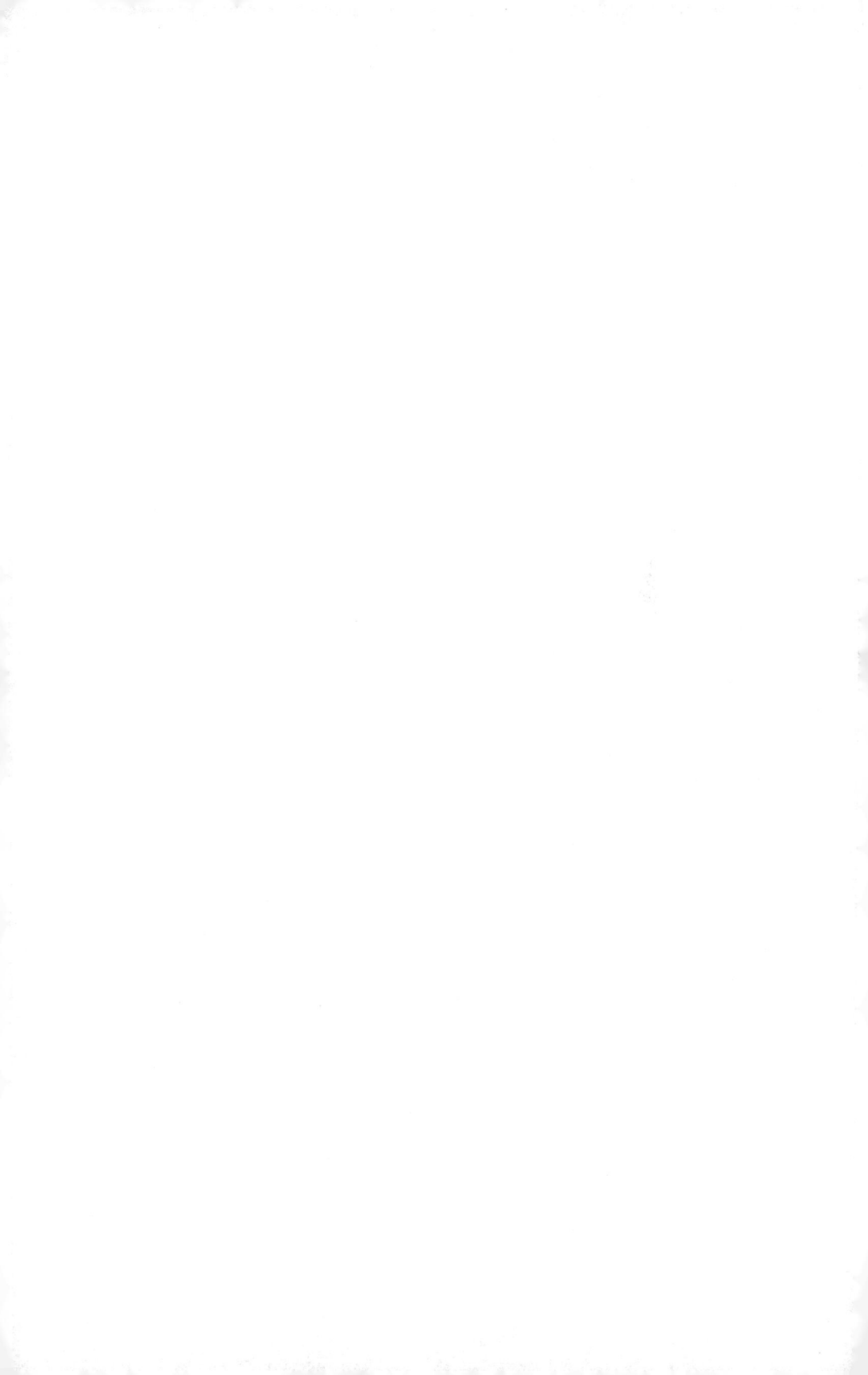

Made in the USA
Columbia, SC
04 June 2021